*The Center for
Contemplative Practice*

shares

YOU KNOW YOU ARE GOING TO DIE, NOW WHAT?

A Lay Cistercian cancer survivor reflects on Three Questions he had to face head-on and how contemplation helped him discover peace, joy and love.

*Participant Workbook
Michael F. Conrad, Ed.D.*

This book is dedicated with grateful affection to three practioners of the healing arts and to the Monastic and Lay Cistercian communites of Our Lady of the Holy Spirit Monastery, Conyers, Ga.

Dr. Scott Tetreault, M.D., Oncologist
Dr. Judith Lewis, M.D. Internal Medicine
Dr. David Tedrick, M.D., Cardiologist

NOTE WELL:
There are four books on How to Die Well. They each have a specific goal.

You Know You Are Going to Die, Now What? How to prepare to live...Forever This is the core book in the series. It gives an in-depth presentation of how to take charge of your life. Do that and death will take care of itself. (240 pages)

You Know You Are Going to Die, Now What? How to prepare to live...Forever: The Workbook. This is an adult education book for parishes on death and dying.

You Know You Are Going to Die, Now What? A Lay Cistercian cancer survivor reflects on Three Questions He Had to Face Head On and how contemplation helped him discover peace, joy and love.
This book is unlike the core book or the workbook. This is a book for parishes and groups to facilitate adult education classes for families who are affected by cancer. It is what I went through when I found out I had cancer and how I used contemplative spirituality as my way to deal with it.

You Know You Are Going to Die, Now What? A cancer survivor reflects on three questions you must face head on: A journal. This is a journal book for you to jot down your ideas and to reflect on three questions that you might be avoiding because they are uncomfortable.

> This book may not be reproduced by photocopying
> without the permission in writing from the publisher.
>
> The Center for Contemplative Practice
> 2402 Glenshire Lane, Tallahassee, FL 32309
>
> Printed in the United States of America
> August, 2017
> Copyright 2017, All Rights Reserved

This book is a workbook resource for you, your family and possibly your parish, to identify three questions that everyone is afraid to ask. As a cancer survivor of Leukemia, CLL type, I had to answer them and I thought you might like the group approach that helps you talk about cancer, what to do if you have it, and what comes next. It is meant to discuss questions in groups of four or five.

Whether you have some faith system or no faith system at all, you have a value system, know it or not. That is your default system of what you hold as your center. Only you can choose what you place at your center, be it money, fame, fortune and glory (as Indiana Jones said in The Temple of Doom) or nothing at all. Before you accuse me of flying false colors, I will tell you that I am a Lay Cistercian (Trappist) member of Our Lady of the Holy Spirit in Conyers, GA. Although it has influenced my view of reality, I am not trying to make you this or that. I don't care. I do care about contemplative practices of silence and solitude and the conversion of my life to the purpose I have selected. I do care to share with you some reflections on how contemplation helped me secure a North on my compass when I learned I had cancer. I hope that you can apply at least one or two ideas to your situation, given that you know you are going to die soon. I do care that you have an opportunity to write down YOUR thoughts and feelings as you confront yourself and the situation in which you find yourself.

There are three questions that I asked myself, upon learning that I had cancer. I used contemplation (going into the rich interior of my inner self) to seek peace, purpose and forgiveness, all within the silence of my own heart. While it is true that you are diagnosed with cancer, or some other life-threatening illness as an individual, you can be sure you don't have it alone, as soon as you allow your friends to share in your diagnosis and assimilate it into their way of thinking. Cancer is always a family disease. The first part of this workbook, I will give you my take on the three questions that I faced. It will be similar to the journal book of the same name. I want both books on cancer and contemplation to have the same first part. The second part of this book is a series of three exercises you share with your tabletop mates. https://thecenterforcontemplativepractice.org
–Michael F. Conrad, Ed.D.

THREE QUESTIONS YOU MUST FACE HEAD ON

QUESTION ONE: AM I GOING TO DIE?

Of course you are! This is the big, elephant-in-the-room question for those who have been told they have cancer or AIDS, the so-called question everyone knows but no one wants to talk about. It is classic avoidance and we all do it. After all, who wants to die? Who wants to be told they are going to die? It affects both patients and physicians. Physicians are petrified because they don't know how their patients will accept it; patients are stunned when they hear the "C" word and begin playing an endless loop of doomsday scenarios of "not me" in their minds. Everyone knows he or she is going to die, but many of us are not prepared, when it is ME that is the subject of that discussion.

The question is not, nor will it ever be, "Am I going to die?" Name one person you know who will not die? I received a phone call from my primary physician, Dr. Judith Lewis, M.D., Internal Medicine, one day in September of 2014, stating she had reviewed my WBC count (> 20) and wanted to make an appointment for me with an Oncologist, Dr. Scott Tetreault, M.D., in Tallahassee, FL. She said to me, "You know what we are talking about, don't you?" I said, "Yes. You are telling me I probably have cancer but you want to make sure with a bone-marrow biopsy." I thought it was nice that she called me. I hung up and had no thoughts in my mind, which some say is normal, but I did fall back on my center, the set of values and meaning that give worth to my life.

Each of us has a center of our being, one that we alone can choose, based on what we value as meaningful in our lives to that point. When there is trauma and urgency, such as when you are told you are going to die, prisoners get religion all of a sudden, those about to die, want to confess to a Priest, if they are Catholic, people think of their value system, as their life moves before their eyes. You may have experienced this. If what we have selected as our center is substantial and meaningful, we stand on the solid grounds of our humanity, if our center is like Jell-O, we don't do so well with the news that we are going to die, or we may have cancer.

Here are some lessons I learned about my center and why the news that I probably had Leukemia rested on a solid foundation of meaning for me.

Lesson One: Keep life simple. Your center is the one ground of your being. The default emotions and feelings, when someone says you are going to die, can be like Kubler-Ross' five steps of grief:
    1 - Denial.
    2 - Anger.
    3 - Bargaining.
    4 - Depression. Also referred to as preparatory grieving. ...
    5 - Acceptance.
https://grief.com/the-five-stages-of-grief/ Not all centers are capable of sustaining you as you work your way through these five stages of grief, let alone provide you with what you need to move to the next stage of your life. When I was told that I had cancer, I don't remember being depressed or angry. When I actually found out that I had a football-size mass of CLL cells in my liver, it was not good news. The worst part for me was not the chemotherapy, twelve sessions of at least five hours apiece, or the liver biposy, but the MRI and PET scan. I am severely claustrophobic.
In 1978, when I was a U.S. Army Chaplain, stationed at Ft. Will, OK, I remember viewing a videotape produced by Dr. Morris Massey called You Are What You Were, When. Check out the URL:
http://changingminds.org/explanations/values/values_development.htm
His thinking has proundly nourished and shaped my views of reality, concepts that, as we live out our lives, are shaped by how and where we grew up and re-shaped by traumatic events, Dr. Massey calls significant emotional events. I want to share with you two such events, since it has to do with cancer and how I reacted to it, when I first heard that I probably had it. I related to you how I first heard of my initial concerns from my Internal Medicine physician that I had something that may be cancerous. Notice that wording? Initially, I had no idea what cancer was, nor what kind I might have, or anything about how to treat it. My first thoughts after hearing what my physician initially said was, "That in all things, God be glorified," a quote from St. Benedict of Norcia (c. 520) What I did was use one of my emotional events (hearing that I had cancer) and immediately answered it with another one, i.e., being accepted as a Lay Cistercian at Holy Spirit Monastery (Trappist) in Conyers, Ga.

I thought I didn't see that unusual reaction coming. It did happen and it was immediate, like a hidden strand of DNA popping into action. I did not have feelings of anxiety or depression. It was like someone saying to me while having a cup of coffee together, "What would you do if you knew the world was going to end in five minutes?" and I said, "Finish my coffee and order a refill." I am still trying to rationalize what happened at that moment and why. As time goes on, I realize that I am what I have been, and my future lies in how I have used my contemplative spirituality event to makes decisions that control events that happen to me in the future, in this case, having cancer.

I am reminded of the saying I penned, *"I am not you; you are not me; God is not you; and, most certainly, you are not God."* Simply put, Dr. Massey says you will react to cancer (any type) or any other trauma, with the values that you have from your childhood, unless there is a significant emotional event that causes you to adjust them. I share this with you because I have found, through the contemplative spirituality of love, that I am not limited by the death of the body, or fear of dying. This does not mean you do or should hold the same ideas. I hope it prompts you to look inside you for peace and happiness, even in the face of imminent death so that you can prepare to die well.

Lesson Two: You die by yourself, but you don't die alone. The family goes through the stages of grief with you. If your family sees you as a defenseless victim they will never raise the one question you need to hear about you're dying and what that would mean. Unless someone from the outside (a friend, minister, rabbi or priest) brings this up, it probably won't be addressed. Every time you meet together, there is the great unspoken taboo that needs to be broken. What I learned is it is my death they are talking about, so I must bring up the subject and address it head on. I could not do that unless my ground for walking was concrete and I was in control of my dying well. I don't control that I will die, but I can control how to die well. I had my wife and daughter accompany me to the Oncologist, Dr. Tetreault's office for the results of my tests. I wanted them to know what I know and not begin conjecturing or playing the "what if" game. It worked out well, in terms of them knowing what I know. In terms of the type of lymphoma, it was CLL type and there were a bunch of these cells in my liver the size of a football. I had to have a liver biopsy to see what was going on. Cancer is a family disease. You are all affected.

Lesson 3: Be realistic. The mind is capable of opening up the wonders of the universe to us, but it can also cause us to play games based on conjecture, conspiracies and what is fantasy. Don't play mind games with yourself. My physician told me specifically what I had and what the future was, putting forth treatment options. Here are some ideas I had when thinking about cancer and my future.

- I need to find out what is fact from what is fiction, when it comes to cancer. You don't get all the information you need right away.
- I need to admit that I have cancer, if that is the diagnosis.
- I need to admit that I may die from cancer, but I choose to stress how to live as fully as I can, with my family and friends.
- My treasure in life is with the living not the dead, i.e., things like money or power.
- I need to re-focus on the purpose of my life and practice contemplation on my personal purpose in life daily found in Philippians 2:5. Actually, I am not doing anything now that I did not do before I had my Leukemia diagnosis.
- As strange as it sound, I need to continue to do the spiritual practices I have learned from being a Lay Cistercian. See www.trappist.net/lay-cistercian. They are:
    - Daily Eucharist to keep my spiritual self fed
    - Daily Lectio Divina to keep my inner self energized
    - Daily adoration before the Blessed Sacrament, as practical
    - Daily recitation of the Liturgy of the Hours in common at Good Shephard parish chapel (Office of Readings at 7:40 am, Morning Prayer at 8:00 a.m. and Evening Prayer at 5:00 pm.. except Sunday, in private)
- I need to create a blog page to express my thinking
  See (https:thecenterforcontemplativepractice.org)
- I need to continue to write my spiritual books, so that I can have a purpose in life and keep up my mind active skills and my thinking somewhat logical.in my old age.
- I need to continue to attend the monthly Gathering Meetings at Holy Spirit Monastery with other Lay Cistercians.
- In my way of thinking, prayer is like an ice cube, if you don't keep it frozen, it will return into its natural state--water. It takes work to keep it frozen. It takes energy that is not your own to run the electricity to freeze it. Don't let your ice melt!

The results of doing all these practices are, to my utter astonishment, totally unpredictable and unexpected. I have grown, almost imperceptibly, into a person of inner peace, one who is not flustered by silly, adolescent tantrums of Democrats and Republicans in politics, one who is centered more and more on love with an ever-deeper appreciation of the relationship with God in my contemplation of life. Contemplation means I do not do all the talking, but, in silence and solitude, I just wait for God to speak when He wants. Now that depends on if you see God as real or a figment of someone's overactive imagination. It is your call, only yours. The results of that relationship with the living God is why I did not have a life-stopping reaction to cancer, just a substantial, but temporary jolt, resulting in resignation and peace. My future life is not of this world at all.

SO WHAT?
You may have noticed a few things stand out from my list of future activities.
1. I have changed very little in what I do in life. Granted, I now know that my Leukemia (CLL) is arrested, but I did not know it when I first learned I had the big "C". Life goes on.
2. Perspective is the key for any approach to life. Be you a spiritual person or, not all of us have values that we fall back on in time of trauma. I have tried to share with you some of mine. Look at your center.
3. Medicine will diagnose and heal your body. Values and spirituality will treat how to deal with it.
4. I am moving forward as though I do not have cancer. Moving forward implies there is something out there toward which you head. In my case, it is Omega. See the writings of Teilhard de Chardin, a Jesuit Paleontologist with a way to look at reality that inspired my own thinking. http://teilharddechardin.org/index.php/teilhards-quotes
5. I am preparing for death, not avoiding it. If death is the end for you, face it head on. You can't stop it, nor even delay it. It is as much a part of you as your birth. It simply means the physical and mental reality cease to exist.
6. If death is not the end for you but there is something beyond, face it head on. Whether you have cancer, AIDS, or another terminal illness, the preparation for death will be the same as if you had no disease at all. I did not know that until I was told I had cancer.
7. I have discovered that the best preparation for death, if you know you are going to die, is to live well.

QUESTION 2: What does it mean to die well?

You have just been told that you have cancer. Probably no one has ever told you that you are going to die. If they have done so, it makes no difference. You must take charge of your life, the only one you have, and begin to live, right to the end. All of us have an end.

Talking about death and dying is not at the top of anyone's "to do" list, but you must face it head on. In the first question, I shared some ideas about cancer. This questions deals with the darker, more elusive topic of death and dying, your death and dying, to be precise. The question you have to talk about is, How can I die well? It may not be number one on your hit parade of questions, but I bring this up because that is what happened to me. I was told I had cancer and my mind jumped straight to "I am going to die." I did not say, "Am I going to die?"

In my case, fortunately for me, my default values instinctively kicked in without a moment's notice. I wrote something about that in Question One. The third question, as you may have guessed, is, so now what?

Here are the three questions you must face, head on.
   1. Am I going to die?
   2. What does it mean to die well?
   3. Now what?

Based on my contemplative prayer, the way I access my inner self and the rock solid center of who I am, I hope to become transformed from self to God. Here are some the ideas that came to my mind, when thinking about the question, What Does It Mean to Die Well?

- Dying well to me means I have changed nothing at all about my values or my spiritual practices. My routine is the same. I have the same passion for writing book (such as this one).
- I am existential in my thinking, i.e., I find myself looking for the ontic possibility of the manifestibility of all being, especially pure Being. On my way to church each morning, I see the Sun shine its golden light on the trees of Tallahassee, and I am reminded of how God gives me light by shining His pure energy on me. I don't take the Sun, the trees, grass, or any being for granted any more.
- Martin Buber influenced me with his I/Thou and I/It concepts. Read http://www.iep.utm.edu/buber/#SH2b

QUESTION THREE: Now What?

Once you have been told that you have cancer (not that you are going to die), comes the treatment and results. This might take some time to play out, maybe two to five months or more. Once you have results based on medical facts, you can ask the question, Now What?

If it happens that you are told your case is terminal and there is nothing you can do, you still have the time from this moment to the end. What are you going to do to fill that? As in my case, my cancer is arrested for the moment, so my life continues as it did before but it is now infused with a new urgency to make what time I have to count as meaningful. Before I knew I had CLL type leukemia, I had made out a bucket list of those things I wanted to do before I died. This was due to the fact that I was 74 years old and statistically did not have much more time to go anything.

TO DO LIST OF WHAT YOU CAN DO NOW
1. Create a "to do" list of what you want to do before you die.
I recommend you make such a bucket list, if you have not done so. What are those things and happenings you want to experience before you die. Go ahead and put down the things you would like to do, even if you know that they are going to be impossible to achieve. On my bucket list, I have dropped off many of them, after I new I had leukemia. I think I had ten or eleven of them. Here are some items on my bucket list that I have dropped of and then revised when I joined the Lay Cistercians of Holy Spirit Monastery. I still have them there, but there is no urgency to complete them.

Bucket list BEFORE I became a Lay Cistercian (in no order of importance)
1. Travel to Canada in an RV to fish and snowmobile. A dream.
2. Write books on contemplative practice. In progress.
3. Create and maintain a blog on contemplative practice. In progress.
4. Lobby for Gil Hodges to be in the Hall of Fame. Getting close.
5. Travel to Saint Meinrad School of Theology for my 50th anniversary. Completed with great satisfaction.
6. Travel to Bora Bora to see the sparkling water. A dream.
7. Meet or have lunch with Hillary Rodham Clinton and her husband.
No possibility of reaching this, but I still have Hope.

List after I became a Lay Cistercian:
Seek God in all things and try to emulate the saying of St. Benedict, that in all things, God be glorified. So far, I am a quart low on reaching that, and will be so in my lifetime.

2. Live simply and fiercely.
Life has become so simple for me. I know that my cancer has been arrested, but it makes no difference. My course is set. I do not have the fear to "keep busy" in retirement just to have something to do. The contemplation and Cistercian practices I have begun to learn in the last few years have refined and deepened my center, the core of my being and that from which all my meaning flows. What sounds a bit philosophical and theoretical would not mean horse feathers, were it not for the fact that it works for me. Those who taste and see how good the Lord is know what I mean. Living simply is at the core of what it means to be human. Simply, as I use it, means that I have discovered my purpose in life and I am content to live out that meaning. Fiercely means loving fiercely, loving being the reason we have reason. Ironically, I will never reach a period when I can say I am there, only that I am on the way. Fierce love means loving God with all your heart, your mind and your strength and your neighbor as yourself. This puts reality in perspective for me. When I found out that I had cancer, nothing changed for me because I had already put in place the very values and purpose in life that most people just begin to think about, when they find out they have the "C" word.

3. Take care of your family and friends.
Rather than be the victim of cancer of some terminal illness, embrace it as being part of your destiny. Help others to see you as one who respects and nourishes life, no matter how long or short it may be. No one gets cancer by himself or herself. No one should grieve about having cancer alone. Show your family that you control your destiny, whatever that is. How you approach, death depends on how you approach life and the value you place on it.

4. Grow ever deeper in the world of inner peace and love through relationship with The Master. Contemplative Cistercian spirituality has helped me not only see each day as a glorious exercise in living, but also how all reality fits together, science, philosophy, rational thinking, and spirituality. The Cistercian part means I follow the teaching and councils of Cistercian men and women from the 11th century to now.
See http://www.cistercianpublications.org, and http://trappist.net

You know you are in the spiritual universe, when the physical, mental and spirituality all align and share energy to each other.

Read my series of three books, Spiritual Apes to get a more in-depth approach to how science, psychology and spirituality all complement each other. https://thecenterforcontemplativepractice.org

Reading all of my assumptions and reasons can be like drinking concentrated orange juice. If you know you have cancer, you are up for the challenge.

5. *What will you take with you to Heaven?* If you are one whose very center is that life does not end, then you need to think about what you will take with you to Heaven. A good book? A copy of Handel's Messiah? I suggest to you that you take what is at your center. In my book, You Know You Are Going to Die, Now What?, I wrote a 40 day retreat you can take to help you focus on what to take with you to Heaven. https//thecenterforcontemplativepractice.org

What sounds like a propagandist trying to hawk his wares, is actually my attempt to try to fit the content of 35 books into this one. I wrote all of these books but three of them before I knew I had cancer and that it was arrested. Just wanted you to know that. Here is what I am taking with me. This may sound a bit churchy to those with a different set of assumptions about reality, but they are mine.

- How to love pure energy as much as I am capable while on earth without getting my circuits fried. (Contemplation)
- How to love others around me, especially those with whom I have distaste or hate on and off.
- How to forgive myself and those around me as The Father has forgiven me through Christ's offering.
- How to take what I have threaded with the *Golden Thread* with me to Heaven. My heaven is what I bring with me (without the two-suitcase limit, of course). I had a thought in one of my contemplation sessions that showed me being presented a golden thread. Everything that reminded me of the glory of God in nature and human activity I thread with this *Golden Thread* and I could take this to Heaven with me. I have sunsets I have threaded, family members, friends I have met along the way, music, books I have read, my pets, essentially everything where I recognize the overwhelming love of the Father through the Son by means of the Holy Spirit in life. My list is growing daily and I can take it with me to Heaven.

- In the end, it is all about Hope that the words said to me through the Prophets, the Scriptures, the Church, the Benedictine and Cistercian mothers and fathers through the centuries are true. Life indeed is too short and if I miss the point of why reality is here just for me in this particular time and place, I only get one shot at the truth. There is only one truth in all reality, physical, mental and spiritual universe. What I put at my center is that truth.
- If you don't have such a view of reality and think that death is the end or there is no such thing as Pure Energy, then you should prepare to live out life as though there was no death. Love your family, forgive those with whom you have dissonance and regain resonance, think back on those with whom you have discovered the meaning of love. Celebrate life. You will be one with all living things who are born, live, procreate, find meaning in your life, grow old, then die.
- I want to take my struggle to convert self to God to Heaven. It is precisely the struggle that is so valuable. I set my sights on "doing" Cistercian spirituality with the goal of transforming myself from merely human purpose to the purpose for which I believe I am created, i.e., an adopted son of the Father. I use Cistercian practices repeatedly, with no expectations, so that I can move there by myself. Read Chapter 4 of St. Benedict's Rule in the third part of this book, to get a good idea of the Tools or Good Works. The tools are only a means to an end, not the end itself. Some religions believe that the ultimate disposition of contemplation is nothingness, or Nirvana. In my experience with contemplation, the last step is simply being in the presence of Being. Far from nothingness, it is everything, the totality of all that is, all physical, mental and spiritual universes as one, The One, Omega, or Heaven. It is a person not a state of being. While on earth, I only try to achieve the Tools of Good Works of St. Benedict, I can never reach them consistently and hold on to them. My reach cannot ever exceed my grasp, as the saying goes. You may think me full of seaweed or oozing alien theories. You might be right. You might be wrong. I like to see patterns of spirituality going back from now to Adam and Eve. This is called heritage and I will not give up my heritage for all the tea in China. I keep think I have learned something new and that this is always the end.

We humans like to think we possess the ultimate truth and beat other people up with it. Science knows this is not true, for there is always a discovery that either casts doubt on a finding or substantially deepens our knowledge of where it fits in reality. That is why I put "A Lay Cistercian" cancer victim looks at three questions to face head on" in the title.
These are my values, my reflections, and purpose in life.

- You must look at reality with the sum total of whom you are and who you will become. In reality, everything spiritual is endless, not in terms of time but in its depth of awareness of how everything fits together in Truth. Science and Contemplative Spirituality will one day sit down together like the lion sitting down with the lamb. You will be able to figure out the relationship how the physical universe of time and matter interfaces love as the ultimate energy of Being. We don't yet have a measuring stick for that.
-

6. Sit down with God and have a heart-to-heart talk. What seems like a nonsensical way to approach cancer might be the most powerful of all. It was for me. When I first received the news that I had a football-size mass of CLL cells in my liver, I didn't think about dying, but how I would communicate with God and seek His counsel. Fortunate for me, I had just been accepted as a Novice in the Lay Cistercians of Holy Spirit Monastery (Trappist). Trappists are contemplative men and women who seclude themselves in a monastery in order to focus on seeking God primarily through recitation of the Liturgy of the Hours and Lectio Divina prayer. This is done repeatedly and patiently, and there are no fast answers, no promises of cures, no taking away the fear and the pain. It is by embracing silence, solitude, keeping up with work, praying with fierce love, and being in the presence of others that make my life worthwhile. These are the five Cistercian practices that I have learned. In making these practices part of my daily routine, I have gradually, almost imperceptibly grown in peace and security, inner strength to face the unseen future, and in ever deepening love with all my heart, my soul, and my strength. I am not perfect nor "there" yet. My "there" awaits me after this body no longer houses my spirit, but my spirit will live…Forever. For me, the end is all about the beginning. I hope that the words said to me, through the Prophets, The Master, the Scriptures, the Church, the Benedictine and Cistercian mothers and fathers through the centuries, are true. Life indeed is too short and if I miss the point of why reality is here just for me in this particular time and place, I only get one shot at the truth. There is only one truth in all reality, physical, mental and spiritual universe. What I put at my center is what I think that truth to be. These are my reflections based on my assumptions. I want to share my struggle to convert self to God to Heaven. It is precisely the time I take to struggle that is so valuable. I set my sights on "doing," not complaining.

As I understand it, Cistercian spirituality is all about the goal of transforming myself from merely human purpose to the purpose for which I believe I am created, i.e., an adopted son of the Father. I use Cistercian practices repeatedly with no expectation that, in this lifetime, I can ever reach that goal by myself. Read Chapter 4 of St. Benedict's Rule in the third part of this book, to get a good idea of the Tools for Good Works. The tools are only a means to an end, not the end itself. Some religions believe that the ultimate disposition of contemplation is nothingness, or Nirvana. In my experience with contemplation, the last step is simply being in the presence of Being. Far from nothingness, it is every thingness, the totality of all that is, all physical, mental and spiritual universes as one, The One, Omega, or Heaven. It is a person not a place. While on earth, I only try to achieve the Tools of Good Works of St. Benedict in Chapter 4 of The Rule. I can never reach them. We humans like to think we possess the ultimate truth and beat other people up with it. Science knows this is not true, for there is always a discovery that either casts doubt on a finding or substantially deepens our knowledge of where it fits in reality. That is why I put "A Lay Cistercian cancer victim looks at three questions to face head-on" as the title. There is always a way to go that is deeper in awareness and how all things fit together. Always! For me, it is spiritual. It is my heritage, won at considerable cost by those who have gone before me. I encourage you to look at both visible and invisible reality with the sum total of whom you are and who you will become. In reality, everything spiritual is endless, not in terms of time but in its depth of awareness of how everything fits together in Truth. Science and Contemplative Spirituality will one day sit down together like the lion sitting down with the lamb. We will be able to figure out the relationship of how the physical universe of time and matter interfaces love as the ultimate energy of Being. Right now, we don't yet have a measuring stick for that. All of us are in this big rowboat called earth as we row our way through time, plugging leaks, taking advantage of the North Star for navigation, and having a destination port, whether we know it or not. There is purpose to the physical universe (being), there is purpose to the mental universe (meaning), and there is, for me, purpose to the spiritual universe (perfect, unconditional love). Too theoretical? Maybe! Too much living in La-La Land? I don't think so! I am betting my life on it.

For those whose world view (weltanschauung) is limited to only two universes, and does not include a Supreme Being, or any God stuff, I would recommend you read St. Benedict's Rule, Chapter 4 on the Tools of Good Works each day, as a guide to being fully human. In reading it this Sunday, I was struck by how good these basic prescriptions for spirituality are well suited for anyone who is trying to live a life that is fully human. I urge you to read them and see what you think (taking out the God stuff, of course).

HOW CONTEMPLATION HELPED ME TO FIND PEACE, JOY AND LOVE

I had one of those epiphanies people talk about, in 2007. You know, a significant emotional event, as Morris Massey would say. I was sitting at my desk at Florida Department of Children and Families, Tallahassee, Florida, when I felt strange (more so than usual) and told someone I thought I would go home a rest awhile. Having retired in 2006, I was doing work in training administration but not as an employee. My friends encouraged me to call 911, since I had pains in my chest and my breathing was labored. Being the pseudo-macho man that I am, I brushed off the suggestion as well meaning. I decided to call 911 and that turned out to be a lifesaver. I had never called 911 before. I got on the stretcher and they put the oxygen mask on me and gave me some nitro pills. I remember looking up at the trees passing by, thinking this is a great ride, and I am glad I called 911. That is all I remembered until I woke up in the Cardiac Intensive Care unit at Tallahassee Memorial Hospital. Later, I was told that as I arrived in the emergency room, my heart stopped. I was revived and taken to a

Cardiac surgical unit where they placed a stint in the blood vessel that comes down over the top of my heart. I had experienced cardiac arrest called "the Widowmaker". It has less than a 10% survival rate. I was in the hospital for a total of four days. That was my first experience with being close to death. Actually, you can say I came back from the dead. Later, I was told that I had a 100% blockage in that artery, and 90% in another one. I ended up with two stents. That was back in 2007, and except for taking lots of pills to keep plaque at bay, I am reasonably healthy.

Back in 2007, I was not aspiring to be a Lay Cistercian, but I don't remember being preoccupied with thinking about dying or the narrow escape that I just experienced with the Grim Reaper. However, it was a wakeup call for me, one that inspired me, in hindsight, to pursue a contemplative approach to reality and my life. It is strange how these major events all think together, although I did not see their connection until much later (a few years ago).

Both of these life-threatening events of the past ten years have funneled me into a contemplative lifestyle. Here is how Cistercian practices have helped me find peace, joy and love within me.
The five practices are:
- Silence
- Solitude
- Work
- Prayer
- Community

I offer my own reflections on these five contemplative practices and how each of them helped me find peace, joy, and love, despite my cardiac arrest and cancer diagnosis. Here is the table, eat what you will.

SILENCE – In order to seek God, you must first put yourself in His presence. That is hard to do, when you first know you have cardiac arrest or cancer, and maybe even impossible. There are so many emotions swirling around in your mind. Eventually the merry-go-round slows down a bit to enable you to accept other concepts and ideas. That is what happened to me, when I was told by someone in the Emergency Room (ER), that, when I arrived at the hospital unconscious, that I had cardiac arrest. Dr. Tedrick, M.D. performed a cardiac catheterization on my LAD and put in a stent. He literally saved my life, for which I am eternally grateful, and I do mean eternally. There is a 10% survival rate on this type of cardiac arrest. https://myheart.net/articles/the-widowmaker/

When I finally woke up, a friend, who visited me in the Cardiac Intensive Care Unit (CICU), asked if I saw any heavenly bright lights while I was out. I told him that all I saw was darkness, so I must have gone to that place of darkness. Looking back on it, I remember I experienced a great sense of peace and joy. That may mean I was given a respite to come back and do some more good, or it could just be that tasted a little of what awaited me.

I bring this up at all because the shock of the illness put me in a state of numbness to all things spiritual. Here is the ironic thing. I did not have to think about my spiritual life. It evidently had defaulted in this emergency to my purpose, my will to live. I had a purpose to live that was not dependent on my spouse, daughter, friends my monetary treasures, or even my job. My center, my purpose for being, was, and is, anchored in the saying from Philippians 2:5, "Have in you the mind of Christ Jesus." What probably sounds too churchy is actually the source of my peace, joy and love. You get to choose your own center, on which you will fall back when you are told you have cancer and may not live a natural life for much longer.

Is your center going to sustain you in time of distress? Will it give you the ability to perceive peace, joy and love, not as the world sees them, but to sit next to God as on a park bench as a friend, together in silence, and soak in pure energy? Choose wisely! It is that energy, outside of myself, that enables me to find a North on my compass and a port during the perfect storms of life

Now, I just say a tiny prayer for God to sit down with me, and then wait. As I become more accustomed to how God speaks to me, I am receiving more insights, such as writing all these books. Where do these ideas come from? I have no idea, except before my *contemplatio*, I had no ideas, and now I can't write them down fast enough. It also helps that I refuse to listen or watch national news with the sophomoric and adolescent fratricide between Democrats and Republicans.

Here are some ideas I have learned about contemplative silence.
- Silence means I talk less and listen more.
- Silence means I do not have to do anything but be open to everything.
- Silence means I do what the results of my listening dictate.
- Silence means I realize that God speaks to me when He wants, not when it is convenient for me.
- Silence means there is a one to One meeting of minds, spirits, and wills. (Did you catch the nuance of the One?)
- Silence is the language of God., not French, English, or any other form of communication. It's outcome is peace, joy, and love.

Why would silence be God's communication, when silence is all about the absence of sound? In one sense, silence means the lack of noise or sounds. We humans communicate with sounds. We call it language. Not everyone can understand the sounds we make to each other. I don't know the Russian language, so someone speaking Russian can't communicate with me, or vice versa.

What language does God speak were it not silence? Remember, God has neither human body nor vocal chords. God speaks through being God. To be in the presence of God is to receive His energy.

Christ, having both divine and human nature, is the bridge between the silence of God and the mind of man. He taught us how to listen to the will of God in our hearts and minds by going to the Father, through, with and in Him, in union with the Holy Spirit. We call that prayer, for lack of a better word.

I see the silence of God as the invisible energy that permeates all time and matter. In contemplative silence, I can tune in to that frequency to receive pure energy, as I am able to receive it through Christ, my transistor, but not without focus and work.

Language is what I use to communicate, namely English. Silence is what God uses to communicate with me. I must know how to speak silence. Contemplation helps with that, more and more, as time goes on.

Silence means there are no words necessary to communicate. Contemplative prayer means I go inside myself through silence and solitude to just stand there and wait to experience (contemplation is a feeling) the presence or energy of God. It is I who must approach God, with a humble and contrite heart, to receive whatever God wills.

It is in this silence of contemplation that I have found a peace that the hectic world can never afford me. This peace is a person that says, and keeps on saying, to me, "Don't be afraid." I don't respond back, just wait, for whatever, or more properly, whoever approaches. I don't have an image of an old man in white beard, sitting on a throne, surrounded by thousands of angels singing His praise. My image is a feeling of fierce love, of pure peace. The only time I have come close to that feeling is when I attended the Morning Prayer (Matins) at Holy Spirit Monastery, Conyers, Ga., at 4:00 a.m. I must tell you that this feeling (contemplatio) did not last long, nor could I sustain it as hard as I tried. I caught only a glimpse of what is my destiny, and I may not ever reach it again, although I will try to love my all my heart and mind and strength, every day. This is why, even though I am tempted every day to put my hope in doing anything to live longer, I am at peace with my heart problems and cancer. After all, what is the loss of the body compared to what the soul gains in peace and joy? There is only one place you can get it. It is totally free for the asking.

If you have cancer or some other life-threatening illness, you have silence, which leads to peace, joy and love, if you access it. Just shut your eyes and focus on listening with your whole being, not just your senses. Now wait.

SOLITUDE: Carving out a space in which to do silent contemplation is not easy, but it is easier than you might think. Look around you for opportunities to be silent, even if there is a lot of noise. I do a lot of contemplation in solitude when I am at Trader Joe's Grocery, or waiting outside Publix. Solitude does not cure cancer, but it can provide a place of safety within you so that you can begin to deal with an even more important reality, now what?

WORK: As someone who has both cancer and cardiac arrest, work means keeping my mind and heart busy. I can putter around the lawn or write books, since I am retired. Work means keeping my mind and

Heart busy. Notice I said my heart. Work is not a job that I have as much as trying to do contemplation and the other practices that lead to peace, joy, and love. That is why I always offer up my morning prayer to sanctify work and whatever I do to, as St. Benedict says, do it for the glory of God. Not a bad way to start a day, don't you think?

PRAY:

Prayer, as I learned it in 6th Grade, is lifting the heart and mind to God. Not much has changed since then, except I now know more of what that means and how to dig beneath the surface to find meaning through both formal and informal prayer..

To pray means at least the following for me.

- Prayer is always performed by an individual, but it is not always private.
- Contemplation is performed by an individual in silence and solitude.
- Prayer is also has a communal aspect. There are not only private prayers, but also public one, such as the Liturgy of the Hours, and Eucharist.
- Prayer is most effective, in my life, when I consistently carve out time for silence and solitude, on a daily basis. It is a habit
- Prayer is the time I take to carve out some space for the one I love and hope to receive a taste of divine energy in return.
  I do my contemplation before the Blessed Sacrament in Eucharistic Adoration, whenever possible.
  http://www.savior.org/devotions.htm

It is before the Blessed Sacrament in contemplation that I found peace, not the peace that comes from knowing that you have cancer and cardiac arrest, but the sustained energy to be beyond it.

COMMUNITY:

As an aspiring Lay Cistercian, community is the crucible, which grinds away my old self and its old ways of thinking and acting, to form a new person. John the Baptist says, "He must increase and I must decrease." This is at the heart of contemplation because contemplation of the One is the intense yearning to sit at the feet of The Master and listen to whatever He says. The more we take up our cross daily and follow The Master, the more we desire to be in that presence. For me, it is the pearl of great price, the sower who sews good seeds, the mustard seed that grows more and more with time, the yeast that mixes with the dough of my life to rise with Christ and make all things new, repeatedly. (Matthew 13) Why? I meet the Holy Spirit in the living Body of Christ, despite the imperfection of its members and my own inadequacies.

- Community prayer means individuals focus their collective minds and hearts on loving God together as one, as Christ is the One.
- Just as you don't have cancer by yourself, you don't pray by yourself, even if you are alone and say informal prayers that you make up.
- Once I die, the community of believers will pray for me that I be loosed from my sins and enter into my inheritance which I hope for doing my journey.
- With my view of reality being that of a community still in the journey and striving for peace for the rest of their lives, those who have died and rest now in peace of The Master, and those who have finished the race but await their reward, those with cancer don't die, even if the body does. Not all agree with this.
- Eucharist is the ultimate collective prayer of the Church because it is not just performed by an individual, or a group of individuals. Each time this prayer is enacted, the whole Church participates, those in Heaven, those still waiting on earth, and those still doing penance in Purgatory.
- The Liturgy of the Hours is a public prayer. The whole Church proclaims the glory of the Father, through the Son, by means of the Holy Spirit. This is done by monastic communities, clergy and laity throughout the world, seven times a day. It has been done since before St. Benedict's time, c. 540 BCE, without interruption, despite the flaws and sinfulness of those praying.
- Prayer is all about communicating with God. Community is all about the product of communicating with God, i.e., practicing the spiritual and corporal works of mercy.
- The Church Universal is the whole assembly of members, those who have died in the Hope of the Resurrection, those still running the race, and those who have not yet completed the course and await their reward.

Community is important for Lay Cistercians because it allows each of us to be Christ bearers to one another using the gifts that we have. For me, this is true even with cancer and cardiac arrest. If you want to be in a community of peace and love, you must practice the contemplative lifestyle with perseverance and persistency. Daily!

THREE QUESTIONS YOU MUST FACE HEAD-ON, IF YOU KNOW YOU ARE GOING TO DIE, AND WHAT TO DO ABOUT IT

NOTA BENE: What follows is a series of three adult learning exercises to help you to design a program to talk about three questions you must face and how contemplation might help you. The purpose of the exercises is to help you talk about cancer or your illness and how you can use contemplation to find peace, joy and love. You may wish to arrange these sessions once a week, or have a mini-retreat on Saturday. You don't have to choose all five for a program. The table is set, choose what you wish to eat.

QUESTION ONE: Am I going to Die?

EXERCISE ONE:

A young minister, flush with the Spirit, rose to address his congregation with these passionate words, "Everyone in this congregation is going to die!" A young woman in the back of the congregation began laughing uncontrollably. Why are you making fun of my statement that all of us in this congregation are going to die?" said the minister, flushed with embarrassment. "I don't belong to this congregation," said the woman.

That woman may not die, but the rest of us will surely die, eventually.

Break into groups of four or five.

Discuss the following statements.
1. Are you going to die? What does that mean, if you do not have cancer? What does it mean if you have been told you have cancer? Is there a difference?
2. Does the fact that you have cancer mean you automatically have a death sentence immediately? Why does having the presence of mind to get all the fact mean so much?
3. If you want life after death, you should make sure that you have life before you die. What does this mean for anyone who knows he or she is going to die?
4. All us have a default position we fall back on in times of trial or major illness. It is called your ground, or your center. What is your center and how can it help you accept the fact that you are going to die?
5. How does humility help you gain perspective on your life?

REFLECTIONS TO CONSIDER:

- Like sex, death is one of those topics that are taboo. Yet it a fact of reality that all of us will not be here one hundred years from now, or so.

- When we confront our worst fears head on, we demystify them, in a way, and make them more acceptable for conversation. Family groups, especially, don't want to be the first one to bring up the "D" word. I have been chastised many times for bring up the possibility of my own death. I accept it, but other don't want to talk about it.

- Fear of death is as old as human recollections. Genesis, that elegant story of why we are who we are, states that we must die but there is hope for the future.

- Spirituality, especially contemplative spirituality that stresses silence, solitude, balance, common sense, work, prayer, and community, is a process that is lasts a lifetime, designed to counter the debilitating effects of original sin.

- We are prone to thinking the worst-case scenario, when we think about cancer.

For me, I had to take some time to change my orientation. By that, I mean *change from thinking about the past;*
- what I would leave behind, when I die,
- what would people do without me?
- and how much I will miss life and love,

to what I will gain in the future;
- what awaits me after I die?
- the fulfillment of all that I have ever done and the meaning I have gained from a lifetime of struggle to be spiritual,
- and my reward of being one with The One, with my family, with my friends and all the threaded realities of my Golden Thread,

…Forever.

QUESTION TWO: How to die well.

EXERCISE:

You won't know how to die well until you have struggled to master, and failed, and keep on trying, how to live well. Life is a process.

If life is all about living well, have you lived well? What does that mean for you? You can either believe that life ends with death, or that life begins with death. Is this statement so much horse feathers? What is the approach you have that would prepare you to accept your cancer and that you are going to die?

Write down three ideas you think about, when you hear the words, "How to die well."

_____
_____
_____
_____

ANSWER THESE QUESTIONS:

In your group, share with each other what you mean by dying well. Be prepared to share two learning points from the discussion.

1. Is thinking about how to die well a waste of time? If so, what you do to prepare yourself for the future, whatever that is.

2. Name three ideas that come to mind when you think of dying well. Are the three ideas ones that you will do, or just talk?

3. Do you find the subject of actually preparing to die well uncomfortable?

4. How would you help a family member, who has cancer, approach the subject of dying well? Would you avoid it?

5. What does "dying with dignity," mean?

REFLECTIONS TO CONSIDER:

What does it mean to be in control of your dying and death? How can you control death? Isn't that impossible? Of course, it is. What you can control is how you approach death by what you do with your life from now until that time comes, and, believe me, it will come for all of us.

Life is all you have, while you still breathe. Don't let life happen to you, like a random roll of the dice in a casino, or a retiree that just watches I Love Lucy reruns to pass the time, until he or she dies.

Find the purpose of life. I found it and use it every day to grow in knowledge, love, and service to my neighbor. My purpose in life is not within me, but the way I access it is, through contemplation and Cistercian charisms and practices. www.trappist.net

In my own case, dying with dignity has to do with being in charge of your last arrangements and getting them lined up, so that family do not have to guess what you want done. My checklist includes: a living will, a last will that is up to date, funeral wishes written down and coordinated with the parish priest and family members, debts identified and paid off, as quickly as possible, all IDs and computer passwords to websites, blogs, etc. written down and gone over with family members. There is actually quite a large laundry list of things to do.

CHECK OUT THE FOLLOWING WEBSITE

www.trappist.com to access eco-burial information from Honey Creek Woodlands Nature Conservancy.

NOW WHAT? You know that you are going to die, now what?

EXERCISE:

Go to a place of solitude and silence and write a poem about your life, your love and your hope for the future. "Now what" is about how you will live your life from this day forward.

Use the space below to write your own poem. Maybe you never wrote a poem before. Great! Whatever you write is fine.

Do this for twenty minutes. Read what I wrote on page 37.

ANSWER THESE QUESTIONS:

Be prepared to share two learning points from the discussion.

1. Those who would like to volunteer to read their poem may do so. (volunteers only). After each reading, discuss the poem in terms of the third question, You Know You Are Going to Die, Now What?

2. How can contemplation and the five Cistercian practices help you to find peace, joy, and love? If not, what will you put in its place to help you with cancer or your terminal illness?

REFLECTIONS TO CONSIDER:

- When you think of these five contemplative practices, don't see them as the world sees them, i.e., limited to meanings based worldly understanding. Rather, see them in the context of a larger reality, helping you confront yourself with cancer or some other life-threatening illness.
- Silence becomes your friend as you face yourself and grow within yourself to discover a new source of energy.
- Solitude becomes an anticipated companion who walks with you as you open yourself up to the totality of all that is.
- Work is a cherished co-worker who guides you and helps you to find meaning and success in contemplation.
- Prayer is the mantel you wear that protects you from the burning rays of the world and keeps you warm, when the cold of despair penetrates your very being.
- Community is joining with others to sing as one, to pray as many, to work together, often in solitude but never alone, all of this in the silence of The One.

Do everything in your power to let your health care professionals focus on your cancer or illness. Do everything in your power to heal your spirit through contact with pure energy. Think again of the purpose of life and where does cancer fit into the center that you chose to live out that purpose.

END NOTES:

The purpose of organizing spiritual practices is not to limit your freedom to contemplate about God but to expand it to encompass the totality of all that is. This is a template to ensure sustainability in practice and consistency of contemplation.

Contemplation, in a manner of speaking, is like a diet. Your physician tells you that you need to lose weight. Now comes the hard part. What diet will you choose, or, if the physician gives you one, will you take it seriously? Based on my own feeble attempts to diet, here are some observations about diets that apply to contemplation.

1. *I won't diet unless my reasons for doing it outweigh my reason for not doing it (laziness).* Cancer, cardiac arrest, and diabetes are three good reasons for me that outweigh not doing it, and even then, I am tempted to take the low road.
2. *No one should diet by themselves.* They need the support from community, family and friends.
3. *I will be tempted, almost every minute, to abandon my goal and eat the forbidden fruit.* Makes you sympathetic with Adam and Eve, don't you think? Doing contemplation is just like that. There is no winning the prize without struggle and practice/failure/practice.
4. *The prize is worth the time you take to master it.* Ask anyone who has lost weight and not gained it back; ask anyone who has even come close to catching a glimpse of the love of Christ through contemplation, and they will tell you.
5. *Failure is not a waste of time, when you try so hard.* What is real failure is losing your will to diet and giving up totally. Because we exists in a condition of original sin (we have to struggle to do what is right), contemplation is not automatic. It takes work, time, and acceptance of our human frailties.
6. *There are many diets out there, all claiming to be "the one" to save you and help you lose weight.* They probably all work. There are many practices out there to help you reach your purpose in life, contemplation being only one of them. To do diets and contemplation justice, you need to perform them consistently and persistently.
7. *Diets are only tools to help you reach your goal.* So too, contemplation is only a methodology to place you in a frame of mind to meet the source of all peace, joy and love.

WEBSITES THAT INCREASE AWARENESS OF THE CONTEMPLATIVE MONK WITHIN EACH OF US

Here are some wonderful, contemplative websites in which you may find some rest for your soul.

http://www.trappist.net

http://www.newadvent.com

https://thecenterforcontemplativepractice.org

https://www.cancer.org/treatment/understanding-yourdiagnosis/talking-about-cancer/listen-with-yourheart/facing-the-final-stage-of-life.html

https://grief.com/

https://siena.org/

http: www.carlmccolman.net

http://www.laycisterciansofgethsemane.org

http://scotthahn.com

http://www.cistercianpublications.org

http://dynamiccatholic.com/

http://www.centeringprayer.com/cntrgpryr.htm

http://www.monk.org

https://cistercianpublications.org/Category/CPCT/Cistercian-Tradition

http://www.saintmeinrad.edu

https://thecenterforcontemplativepractice.org

THE CHRIST IMPERATIVES
LISTEN TO ME, FOR I AM MEEK AND HUMBLE OF HEART.
Matthew 11:28-30

- √ Thirsty? Drink of the living waters! John 7:37.

- √ Hungry? Eat the food that gives eternal life! John 6:33-38.

- √ Bewildered? Believe in the Master! John 3:11-21.

- √ Without hope? Be not afraid! John 13:33-35.

- √ Lost? Find the way. John 14:6-7.

- √ Tired because of the pain? Be renewed! John 15:1-7.

- √ Afraid? Find peace! John 27-28.

- √ Afraid to believe? Believe! John 11:25-27.

- √ Without a family? Listen! John 10:7-18.

- √ In darkness? Walk in the light! John 8:12.

- √ Spiritually depressed? Be healed! John 5:24

Welcome, good and faithful servant, into the Kingdom prepared for you before the world began.

THE CONEMPLATIVE PRACTICE SERIES

SPIRITUAL APES: Our Journey to Forever, Vol. I.

SPIRITUAL APES: Our Journey from Animality to Spirituality, Vol II.

SPIRITUAL APES: The Struggle to Be Spiritual, Vol. III.

HOW TO GRIEVE WELL. What Happens to You When You Have Lost Loved One? Spirituality for the Bereaved.

What Happens to You When You Have Lost a Pet? Spirituality for Pet Owners.

HOW TO DIE WELL. So You Know You Are Going to Die, Now What? A Spiritual Preparation for Life...Forever.

Have You Lost All Your Marbles...or Just Your EX? Spiritual Perspectives for Divorced Women

Searching for Love in the Garden of Eden. Spirituality for the Lonely of Heart.

If Life is a Journey, Have You Lost the Road Map? Spiritual Toolkit for Divorced Men.

Spiritual Estate Planning: Can the Rich Get to Heaven?

Is Your Spiritual Life Running on Empty? Overcoming Spiritual Depression.

Resolving Spiritual Conflicts:101 Ways Split-Religion Moms and Dads Can Agree.

How Moms and Dads Can Be Spiritual Directors: Developmental Spirituality.

Who Does God Think He Is, Anyway? Guidance from the Master.

The Woman Who Changed Time: Spirituality and Time.

You Are My Heritage: A Father's Thoughts as His Daughter Enters College.

17 Skills Moms and Dads Must Teach Their Children: Show Your Children How to Get to Heaven.

Who Rows Your Boat? How to Be Happier Than You Can Possibly Imagine.

Three Rules of the Spiritual Universe: How to Choose an Authentic Center That Leads to Heaven.

Six Thresholds of Life: How to prepare to live…Forever. Participant Workbook.

Facilitating Adult Learning: How to facilitate The Center for Contemplative Practice workshops.

JOURNAL OF MEANING SERIES

Come, Share Your Lord's Joy: A Journal to Prepare for Life...Forever.

Spiritual Estate Planning: A Journal to Build Spiritual Wealth You Can Take to Heaven.

You Are My Heritage: Thoughts on How Much You Mean to Me.

The Center of My Life: Thoughts on the Assumptions Underlying What I Believe.

LAZER LEARNING SERIES

How to Stop Assumicide. How to Think Critically About What You Believer, Without Destroying Your Faith.

Mining for Heavenly Gold While On Earth: How to Center Yourself on What Is Authentic.

Five Steps to Build a Better Future for Your Community: What should your community look like in the future?

Resolving Spiritual Conflicts: Spirituality for Split-Religion Moms and

ADULT LEARNING WORKBOOK SERIES

HOW TO DIE WELL: You know you are going to die, now what? Tabletop Exercises for Facilitators in Adult Learning Centers, Book One

HOW TO GRIEVE WELL: What happens to you when you have lost a loved one? Tabletop Exercises for Facilitators in Adult Learning Centers,

You Know You Are Going to Die, Now What? A Lay Cistercian cancer survivor reflects on three questions you must face head on. The Workbook.

You Know You Are Going to Die, Now What? A Lay Cistercian cancer survivor reflects on three questions you must face head on: A Journal.

WHAT IS THE CENTER FOR CONTEMPLATIVE PRACTICE?

The Center for Contemplative Practice is a ministry of people devoted to providing spiritual resources for adults, such as publishing books, retreats, training, blogs, and on-line meditations.

DISCLAIMER

The ideas and meditations contained in any books or blogs shared by The Center for Contemplative Practice do not represent the official, authoritative teaching of the Roman Catholic Church or any Cistercian Monastery or Lay Cistercian group. These ideas and are the results of *lectio divina* spiritual meditations by the author and reflect only his interpretation of Catholic spiritual thoughts through contemplation

ABOUT THE AUTHOR

Michael F. Conrad, B.S., M.R.E., Ed.D., is retired from a full life of trying to make money, seek fame and recognition by the world, all without much success. Coming to his senses, even after the age of 70, he now struggles to have in him the mind of Christ Jesus. (Philippians 2:5-12) Still running the race and searching for the prize, he has had a lifetime of activities to help him in his quest: he is proud to have been a U.S. Army Chaplain, pastor of parish ministry, adjunct instructor of Adult Education at Indiana University (Bloomington) and University of South Florida (Tampa) and Barry University (Florida), high school instructor of religion, trainer of managers and supervisors, adjunct trainer for the Florida Certified Public Manager program, instructional designer for the State of Florida, former Florida Supreme Court Certified Family Mediator, and currently a publisher, blogger and author, He is a Lay Cistercian member of Our Lady of the Holy Spirit Monastery, Conyers, Georgia, proud father of a daughter, and a humbled husband.

My Life as a Poem

I sing the song of life and love...
    ...sometimes flat and out of tune
    ...sometimes eloquent and full of passion
    ...sometimes forgetting notes and melody
    ...sometimes quaint and intimate
    ...often forgetful and negligent
    ...often in tune with the very core of my being
    ...often with the breath of those who would pull me down, shouting right in my face that I am no good
    ...often with the breath of life uplifting me to heights never before dreamed
    ...greatly grateful for the gift of humility and obedience to The One
    ...greatly thankful for adoption, discovery of a new life of pure energy
    ...greatly appreciative for sharing meaning with others of The Master
    ...greatly sensitive for not judging the motives of anyone but me
    ...happy to be accepted as an aspiring Lay Cistercian
    ...happy to spend time in Eucharistic Adoration
    ...happy and humbled to be an adopted son of the Father
    ...happy for communities of faith and love with wife, daughter, and friends
    ...mindful that the passage of time increases each year
    ...mindful of the major distractions of cancer and cardiac arrest
    ...mindful of my center and the perspective that I am loved and must love back with all the energy of my heart and strength, yet failing
    ...mindful the energy I receive from The One in Whom I find purpose and meaning...Forever.

To The One who is, Who was, and Who is to come at the end of the ages, be glory, honor, power and blessings through The Redeemer Son in unity with the Advocate, Spirit of Love.

From The One who is, Who was, and Who is to come at the end of the ages, I seek hope that His words about the purpose of life are true, that He is the way that leads me to life...Forever.

With The One who is, Who was, and Who is to come at the end of the ages, I seek His fierce love so I can have in me the mind of Christ Jesus, my personal purpose in life and my center...Forever.

"That in all things, may God be glorified." –St. Benedict

MORNING OFFERING PRAYER

Our Father, we offer to you all our thoughts and actions this day, in union with the Sacred Heart of Jesus, in reparation for our sins, and in the hope of the resurrection.

May the work we do today, help us to love you with all our minds and all our hearts, glorify you through your Son, Jesus Christ, by the working of the Holy Spirit. Amen

That in all things, God be glorified. -St. Benedict

www.ingramcontent.com/pod-product-compliance
Lightning Source LLC
Chambersburg PA
CBHW031557210526
45464CB00003B/1326